PLANT-BASED RECIPES FOR DIABETIC KIDNEY DISEASE

A collection of mouth-watering recipes that are both healthy and satisfying, perfect for people with diabetes and kidney disease.

Dr Lily Morgan

COPYRIGHT PAGE

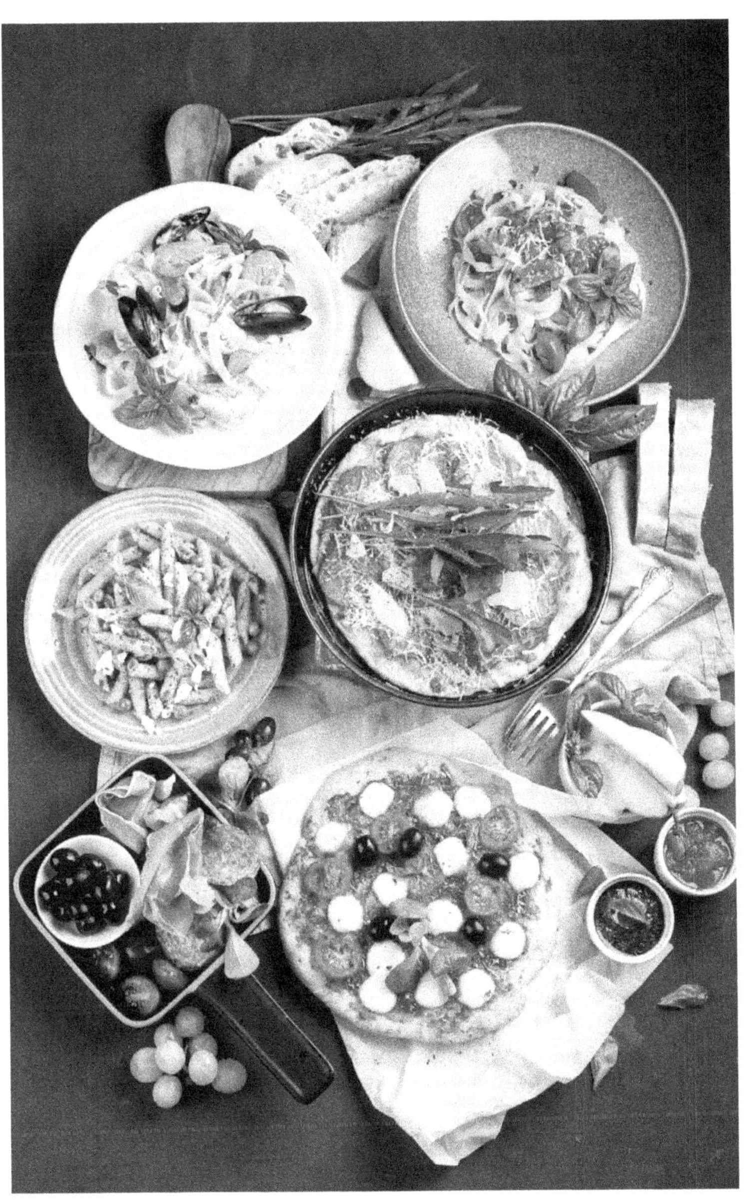

TABLE OF CONTENTS

Chapter 5: Snacks and Appetizers 72

Chapter 6: Desserts 89

Chapter 7: Smoothies 106

INTRODUCTION

I n today's fast-paced world, where health issues are on the rise, understanding the importance of nutrition and its impact on our well-being has become increasingly crucial. One such health concern that demands attention is Diabetic Kidney Disease (DKD). This condition arises when diabetes damages the kidneys, leading to impaired kidney function over time. Managing DKD requires a thoughtful and strategic approach to diet and lifestyle.

In this chapter, we will delve deep into the world of plant-based nutrition and its potential to alleviate the challenges posed by Diabetic Kidney Disease. We will explore the underlying principles behind a plant-based diet and how it can promote better kidney health and overall well-being.

Understanding Diabetic Kidney Disease

Diabetic Kidney Disease, also known as diabetic nephropathy, is a common complication of diabetes. As blood sugar levels remain consistently high over an extended period, the delicate blood vessels in the kidneys become damaged. Over time, this damage impairs the kidneys' ability to filter waste and excess fluids from the blood, leading to a build-up of toxins and potential fluid retention.

The consequences of uncontrolled DKD can be severe, including chronic kidney disease (CKD) and even end-stage renal disease (ESRD), necessitating dialysis or kidney transplant. Therefore, managing DKD and preventing its progression is of utmost importance.

Benefits of a Plant-based Diet for Diabetic Kidney Disease

Research has shown that a well-balanced plant-based diet can be highly beneficial for individuals with Diabetic Kidney Disease. Let's explore some of the key advantages:

Blood Sugar Management: A plant-based diet that focuses on whole foods and minimizes refined sugars can contribute to better blood sugar control, which is vital for managing diabetes and reducing the strain on the kidneys.

Lowering Blood Pressure: Hypertension is a common complication of DKD. Plant-based diets, rich in potassium and low in sodium, have been associated with lower blood pressure levels, potentially easing the burden on the kidneys.

Kidney Function Support: Certain plant-based foods, such as leafy greens and berries, contain antioxidants and anti-inflammatory properties that may support kidney health and function.

Heart Health: A plant-based diet is often heart-friendly, as it tends to be low in saturated fats and cholesterol. Improved cardiovascular health indirectly benefits kidney health as well.

Weight Management: Plant-based diets are generally lower in calories, which can aid in weight management. Maintaining a healthy weight is essential for individuals with DKD, as obesity can worsen kidney function.

Lowering Protein Intake: In advanced stages of DKD, reducing protein intake may be beneficial to lessen the strain on the kidneys. Plant-based diets can offer protein from sources that are gentler on the kidneys.

Tips for Meal Planning and Preparation

Transitioning to a plant-based diet can seem daunting, but with the right approach, it can be a rewarding and enjoyable journey. Here are some practical tips for meal planning and preparation:

Gradual Transition: If you're new to plant-based eating, consider making the shift gradually. Start by incorporating more fruits, vegetables, and whole grains into your meals while reducing animal-based products slowly.

Variety is Key: Embrace the diversity of plant-based foods. Experiment with different grains, legumes, vegetables, fruits, nuts, and seeds to keep your meals exciting and nutrient-rich.

Protein Balance: Ensure you're getting an adequate amount of protein from plant-based sources such as tofu, tempeh, lentils, chickpeas, quinoa, and nuts. Balancing protein intake is essential for kidney health.

Mindful Cooking Methods: Opt for cooking methods that preserve nutrients while minimizing added fats and sodium. Steaming, baking, roasting, and sautéing with minimal oil are excellent choices.

Hydration: Staying well-hydrated is crucial for kidney health. Drink plenty of water throughout the day to support kidney function and flush out toxins.

By incorporating these tips into your daily life, you can embark on a path towards improved kidney health and overall well-being with the power of plant-based nutrition. In the following chapters, we will provide you with practical and delectable recipes that cater to your taste buds and nourish your body.

As we journey through this book, remember that a well-planned plant-based diet, combined with regular physical activity and mindful lifestyle choices, can offer a new lease of life for individuals living with Diabetic Kidney Disease. Let us now move forward and explore the wonders of plant-based cooking for a healthier tomorrow.

Chapter 1: 30 Day Meal Plan

Week 1:

Day 1:

Breakfast: Hearty Quinoa Porridge with Berries and Almonds

Lunch: Rainbow Veggie and Quinoa Salad with Lemon-Tahini Dressing

Dinner: Creamy Vegan Alfredo with Asparagus and Peas

Snack: Baked Sweet Potato Fries with Smoky Paprika Dip

Dessert: Chocolate Avocado Mousse

Day 2:

Breakfast: Green Smoothie Bowl with Spinach and Chia Seeds

Lunch: Mediterranean Chickpea Salad with Fresh Herbs

Dinner: Eggplant Parmesan with Marinara Sauce and Cashew Cheese

Snack: Zucchini and Carrot Fritters with Mint Yogurt Sauce

Dessert: Berry Crisp with Oat and Almond Topping

Day 3:

Breakfast: Avocado Toast with Cherry Tomatoes and Balsamic Glaze

Lunch: Lentil and Vegetable Soup

Dinner: Moroccan Chickpea Stew with Couscous

Snack: Edamame with Sea Salt and Lime

Dessert: Chia Seed and Mixed Fruit Parfait

Day 4:

Breakfast: Vegan Banana Pancakes with Coconut Yogurt

Lunch: Stuffed Bell Peppers with Brown Rice and Lentils

Dinner: Vegan Mushroom Stroganoff over Brown Rice

Snack: Spicy Buffalo Cauliflower Bites with Vegan Ranch Dip

Dessert: Vegan Lemon Bars with Almond Crust

Day 5:

Breakfast: Tofu Scramble with Bell Peppers and Turmeric

Lunch: Grilled Eggplant and Zucchini Panini with Pesto

Dinner: Thai Green Curry with Tofu and Vegetables

Snack: Guacamole with Baked Tortilla Chips

Dessert: Baked Apples with Cinnamon and Maple Syrup

Day 6:

Breakfast: Sweet Potato and Black Bean Breakfast Burritos

Lunch: Cauliflower Rice Stir-fry with Tofu and Veggies

Dinner: Jackfruit and Black Bean Enchiladas

Snack: Stuffed Mushrooms with Quinoa and Spinach

Dessert: Coconut Mango Rice Pudding

Day 7:

Breakfast: Mixed Berry Chia Seed Pudding

Lunch: Sweet Potato and Black Bean Tacos

Dinner: Ratatouille with Quinoa

Snack: Cucumber, Radish, and Vegan Cream Cheese Tea Sandwiches

Dessert: Pumpkin Spice Energy Bites

Week 2

Day 8:

Breakfast: Oatmeal with Cinnamon, Apples, and Walnuts

Lunch: Spinach and Mushroom Quiche with a Chickpea Flour Crust

Dinner: Spicy Peanut Noodles with Broccoli and Tofu

Snack: Roasted Chickpeas with Rosemary and Sea Salt

Dessert: Chocolate Chip Chickpea Blondies

Day 9:

Breakfast: Coconut and Mango Overnight Oats

Lunch: Cucumber and Avocado Sushi Rolls

Dinner: Baked Falafel with Hummus and Tabouli

Snack: Salsa Verde with Homemade Pita Chips

Dessert: Vegan Carrot Cake with Cashew Cream Frosting

Day 10:

Breakfast: Blueberry Buckwheat Muffins

Lunch: Greek-style Lemon Potatoes with Roasted Asparagus

Dinner: Coconut Red Lentil Dahl with Basmati Rice

Snack: Marinated Olives and Artichoke Hearts

Dessert: Frozen Banana and Berry Popsicles

Day 11:

Breakfast: Hearty Quinoa Porridge with Berries and Almonds

Lunch: Rainbow Veggie and Quinoa Salad with Lemon-Tahini Dressing

Dinner: Creamy Vegan Alfredo with Asparagus and Peas

Snack: Baked Sweet Potato Fries with Smoky Paprika Dip

Dessert: Chocolate Avocado Mousse

Day 12:

Breakfast: Green Smoothie Bowl with Spinach and Chia Seeds

Lunch: Mediterranean Chickpea Salad with Fresh Herbs

Dinner: Eggplant Parmesan with Marinara Sauce and Cashew Cheese

Snack: Zucchini and Carrot Fritters with Mint Yogurt Sauce

Dessert: Berry Crisp with Oat and Almond Topping

Day 13:

Breakfast: Avocado Toast with Cherry Tomatoes and Balsamic Glaze

Lunch: Lentil and Vegetable Soup

Dinner: Moroccan Chickpea Stew with Couscous

Snack: Edamame with Sea Salt and Lime

Dessert: Chia Seed and Mixed Fruit Parfait

Day 14:

Breakfast: Vegan Banana Pancakes with Coconut Yogurt

Lunch: Stuffed Bell Peppers with Brown Rice and Lentils

Dinner: Vegan Mushroom Stroganoff over Brown Rice

Snack: Spicy Buffalo Cauliflower Bites with Vegan Ranch Dip

Dessert: Vegan Lemon Bars with Almond Crust

Week 3

Day 15:

Breakfast: Tofu Scramble with Bell Peppers and Turmeric

Lunch: Grilled Eggplant and Zucchini Panini with Pesto

Dinner: Thai Green Curry with Tofu and Vegetables

Snack: Guacamole with Baked Tortilla Chips

Dessert: Baked Apples with Cinnamon and Maple Syrup

Day 16:

Breakfast: Sweet Potato and Black Bean Breakfast Burritos

Lunch: Cauliflower Rice Stir-fry with Tofu and Veggies

Dinner: Jackfruit and Black Bean Enchiladas

Snack: Stuffed Mushrooms with Quinoa and Spinach

Dessert: Coconut Mango Rice Pudding

Day 17:

Breakfast: Mixed Berry Chia Seed Pudding

Lunch: Sweet Potato and Black Bean Tacos

Dinner: Ratatouille with Quinoa

Snack: Cucumber, Radish, and Vegan Cream Cheese Tea
Sandwiches

Dessert: Pumpkin Spice Energy Bites

Day 18:

Breakfast: Oatmeal with Cinnamon, Apples, and Walnuts

Lunch: Spinach and Mushroom Quiche with a Chickpea
Flour Crust

Dinner: Spicy Peanut Noodles with Broccoli and Tofu

Snack: Roasted Chickpeas with Rosemary and Sea Salt

Dessert: Chocolate Chip Chickpea Blondies

Day 19:

Breakfast: Coconut and Mango Overnight Oats

Lunch: Cucumber and Avocado Sushi Rolls

Dinner: Baked Falafel with Hummus and Tabouli

Snack: Salsa Verde with Homemade Pita Chips

Dessert: Vegan Carrot Cake with Cashew Cream Frosting

Day 20:

Breakfast: Blueberry Buckwheat Muffins

Lunch: Greek-style Lemon Potatoes with Roasted Asparagus

Dinner: Coconut Red Lentil Dahl with Basmati Rice

Snack: Marinated Olives and Artichoke Hearts

Dessert: Frozen Banana and Berry Popsicles

Day 21:

Breakfast: Hearty Quinoa Porridge with Berries and Almonds

Lunch: Rainbow Veggie and Quinoa Salad with Lemon-Tahini Dressing

Dinner: Creamy Vegan Alfredo with Asparagus and Peas

Snack: Baked Sweet Potato Fries with Smoky Paprika Dip

Dessert: Chocolate Avocado Mousse

Week 4

Day 22:

Breakfast: Green Smoothie Bowl with Spinach and Chia Seeds

Lunch: Mediterranean Chickpea Salad with Fresh Herbs

Dinner: Eggplant Parmesan with Marinara Sauce and
Cashew Cheese

Snack: Zucchini and Carrot Fritters with Mint Yogurt
Sauce

Dessert: Berry Crisp with Oat and Almond Topping

Day 23:

Breakfast: Avocado Toast with Cherry Tomatoes and
Balsamic Glaze

Lunch: Lentil and Vegetable Soup

Dinner: Moroccan Chickpea Stew with Couscous

Snack: Edamame with Sea Salt and Lime

Dessert: Chia Seed and Mixed Fruit Parfait

Day 24:

Breakfast: Vegan Banana Pancakes with Coconut Yogurt

Lunch: Stuffed Bell Peppers with Brown Rice and Lentils

Dinner: Vegan Mushroom Stroganoff over Brown Rice

Snack: Spicy Buffalo Cauliflower Bites with Vegan Ranch
Dip

Dessert: Vegan Lemon Bars with Almond Crust

Day 25:

Breakfast: Tofu Scramble with Bell Peppers and Turmeric

Lunch: Grilled Eggplant and Zucchini Panini with Pesto

Dinner: Thai Green Curry with Tofu and Vegetables

Snack: Guacamole with Baked Tortilla Chips

Dessert: Baked Apples with Cinnamon and Maple Syrup

Day 26:

Breakfast: Sweet Potato and Black Bean Breakfast Burritos

Lunch: Cauliflower Rice Stir-fry with Tofu and Veggies

Dinner: Jackfruit and Black Bean Enchiladas

Snack: Stuffed Mushrooms with Quinoa and Spinach

Dessert: Coconut Mango Rice Pudding

Day 27:

Breakfast: Mixed Berry Chia Seed Pudding

Lunch: Sweet Potato and Black Bean Tacos

Dinner: Ratatouille with Quinoa

Snack: Cucumber, Radish, and Vegan Cream Cheese Tea Sandwiches

Dessert: Pumpkin Spice Energy Bites

Day 28:

Breakfast: Oatmeal with Cinnamon, Apples, and Walnuts

Lunch: Spinach and Mushroom Quiche with a Chickpea
Flour Crust

Dinner: Spicy Peanut Noodles with Broccoli and Tofu

Snack: Roasted Chickpeas with Rosemary and Sea Salt

Dessert: Chocolate Chip Chickpea Blondies

Day 29:

Breakfast: Coconut and Mango Overnight Oats

Lunch: Cucumber and Avocado Sushi Rolls

Dinner: Baked Falafel with Hummus and Tabouli

Snack: Salsa Verde with Homemade Pita Chips

Dessert: Vegan Carrot Cake with Cashew Cream Frosting

Day 30:

Breakfast: Blueberry Buckwheat Muffins

Lunch: Greek-style Lemon Potatoes with Roasted
Asparagus

Dinner: Coconut Red Lentil Dahl with Basmati Rice

Snack: Marinated Olives and Artichoke Hearts

Dessert: Frozen Banana and Berry Popsicles

Chapter 2: Breakfast Recipes

When it comes to starting the day on a wholesome note, breakfast is the key. For those following a plant-based diet and managing diabetic kidney disease, these breakfast recipes are not only delicious but also packed with nutrition to keep you energized throughout the day.

Hearty Quinoa Porridge with Berries and Almonds

Ingredients:

- 1/2 cup quinoa, rinsed
- 1 cup unsweetened almond milk
- 1/2 cup mixed berries (blueberries, strawberries, raspberries)
- 2 tablespoons sliced almonds
- 1 tablespoon maple syrup
- 1/2 teaspoon vanilla extract
- Pinch of salt

Instructions:

1. In a saucepan, combine quinoa, almond milk, and a pinch of salt. Bring it to a boil.

2. Reduce heat to low, cover, and let it simmer for 15-20 minutes or until quinoa is cooked and liquid is absorbed.

3. Stir in the maple syrup and vanilla extract.

4. Transfer the porridge to serving bowls and top with mixed berries and sliced almonds.

5. Drizzle a little extra maple syrup if desired. Enjoy!

Green Smoothie Bowl with Spinach and Chia Seeds

Ingredients:

- 2 cups baby spinach leaves
- 1 frozen banana
- 1/2 cup frozen mango chunks
- 1 tablespoon chia seeds
- 1 cup unsweetened almond milk
- Fresh fruit slices and nuts for topping (optional)

Instructions:

1. In a blender, combine baby spinach, frozen banana, frozen mango, chia seeds, and almond milk.
2. Blend until smooth and creamy.
3. Pour the green smoothie into a bowl.
4. Top with fresh fruit slices and nuts for added texture and flavor.
5. Enjoy this vibrant and nutrient-packed green smoothie bowl!

Avocado Toast with Cherry Tomatoes and Balsamic Glaze

Ingredients:

- 2 slices whole-grain bread, toasted
- 1 ripe avocado, pitted and mashed
- Cherry tomatoes, halved
- Balsamic glaze
- Fresh basil leaves (optional)
- Salt and pepper to taste

Instructions:

1. Spread the mashed avocado evenly on the toasted bread slices.

2. Top with halved cherry tomatoes and fresh basil leaves (if using).

3. Drizzle balsamic glaze over the toppings.

4. Sprinkle a pinch of salt and pepper for seasoning.

5. Indulge in the creamy, savory goodness of avocado toast!

Vegan Banana Pancakes with Coconut Yogurt

Ingredients:

- 1 cup all-purpose flour
- 2 tablespoons coconut sugar
- 2 teaspoons baking powder
- 1/4 teaspoon salt
- 1 cup unsweetened almond milk
- 1 ripe banana, mashed
- 1 teaspoon vanilla extract
- Coconut oil for greasing the pan

Instructions:

1. In a bowl, whisk together flour, coconut sugar, baking powder, and salt.
2. In a separate bowl, mix almond milk, mashed banana, and vanilla extract.
3. Combine the wet and dry ingredients until just combined. Do not overmix; lumps are okay.
4. Heat a non-stick skillet over medium heat and grease it with coconut oil.
5. Pour 1/4 cup of batter onto the skillet for each pancake.
6. Cook until bubbles appear on the surface, then flip and cook the other side until golden brown.
7. Serve the fluffy vegan banana pancakes with a dollop of coconut yogurt on top.

Tofu Scramble with Bell Peppers and Turmeric

Ingredients:

- 1 block firm tofu, drained and crumbled
- 1/2 red bell pepper, diced

- 1/2 green bell pepper, diced
- 1 small onion, diced
- 1 tablespoon nutritional yeast (optional)
- 1 teaspoon ground turmeric
- 1/2 teaspoon garlic powder
- Salt and pepper to taste
- Fresh parsley for garnish (optional)

Instructions:

1. In a pan, sauté diced bell peppers and onions until they soften.
2. Add crumbled tofu to the pan and mix well with the vegetables.
3. Sprinkle ground turmeric, garlic powder, nutritional yeast (if using), salt, and pepper over the tofu mixture.
4. Continue cooking for another 3-5 minutes until the tofu absorbs the flavors and resembles scrambled eggs.
5. Garnish with fresh parsley for an extra touch of freshness.
6. Enjoy this protein-packed and savory tofu scramble!

Sweet Potato and Black Bean Breakfast Burritos

Ingredients:

- 2 large sweet potatoes, peeled and diced
- 1 can black beans, drained and rinsed
- 1 teaspoon ground cumin
- 1/2 teaspoon chili powder
- Salt and pepper to taste
- Whole-grain tortillas
- Avocado slices (optional)
- Fresh cilantro for garnish (optional)

Instructions:

1. Steam or boil the diced sweet potatoes until tender.
2. In a pan, combine the cooked sweet potatoes and black beans.
3. Add ground cumin, chili powder, salt, and pepper to the pan and mix well.
4. Warm the whole-grain tortillas and spoon the sweet potato and black bean mixture onto each tortilla.
5. Top with avocado slices and fresh cilantro (if using).

6. Roll up the burritos and serve them for a satisfying and hearty breakfast.

Mixed Berry Chia Seed Pudding

Ingredients:

- 1/4 cup chia seeds
- 1 cup unsweetened almond milk
- 1 tablespoon maple syrup
- 1/2 teaspoon vanilla extract
- Mixed berries (blueberries, strawberries, raspberries)

Instructions:

1. In a bowl, mix chia seeds, almond milk, maple syrup, and vanilla extract.
2. Stir well to combine all ingredients thoroughly.
3. Refrigerate the mixture for at least 2 hours or overnight to allow the chia seeds to absorb the liquid and form a pudding-like consistency.
4. Before serving, give it a good stir to make sure the chia seeds are evenly distributed.

5. Top with mixed berries for added natural sweetness and color.

6. Relish in the guilt-free pleasure of this delightful mixed berry chia seed pudding!

Oatmeal with Cinnamon, Apples, and Walnuts

Ingredients:

- 1 cup rolled oats
- 2 cups water or unsweetened almond milk
- 1 apple, diced
- 1/4 cup chopped walnuts
- 1 teaspoon ground cinnamon
- 1 tablespoon maple syrup (optional)
- Pinch of salt

Instructions:

1. In a saucepan, bring water or almond milk to a boil.
2. Stir in rolled oats and reduce heat to low. Cook for about 5 minutes, stirring occasionally.

3. Add diced apples, chopped walnuts, ground cinnamon, and a pinch of salt to the oatmeal.

4. Continue cooking for an additional 2-3 minutes until the apples soften and the oats reach the desired consistency.

5. For a touch of sweetness, drizzle with maple syrup (optional).

6. Savor the comforting flavors of cinnamon, apples, and walnuts in this nourishing oatmeal.

Coconut and Mango Overnight Oats

Ingredients:

- 1 cup rolled oats
- 1 cup unsweetened coconut milk
- 1 ripe mango, diced
- 2 tablespoons shredded coconut
- 1 tablespoon maple syrup (optional)

Instructions:

1. In a jar or airtight container, combine rolled oats and coconut milk.

2. Add diced mango and shredded coconut to the jar.

3. Mix all the ingredients thoroughly and seal the jar.

4. Refrigerate the jar overnight or for at least 4 hours to allow the oats to soak and soften.

5. Before serving, give the overnight oats a good stir.

6. If you prefer it sweeter, drizzle with maple syrup (optional).

7. Relish in the tropical goodness of coconut and mango in this easy-to-prep overnight oats.

Blueberry Buckwheat Muffins

Ingredients:

- 1 cup buckwheat flour
- 1/2 cup almond flour
- 1 teaspoon baking powder
- 1/2 teaspoon baking soda
- 1/4 teaspoon salt
- 1/2 cup unsweetened almond milk
- 1/4 cup maple syrup
- 1 ripe banana, mashed
- 1 cup fresh blueberries

Instructions:

1. Preheat your oven to 350°F (175°C) and line a muffin tin with liners.

2. In a large bowl, whisk together buckwheat flour, almond flour, baking powder, baking soda, and salt.

3. In a separate bowl, combine almond milk, maple syrup, and mashed banana.

4. Add the wet ingredients to the dry ingredients and mix until just combined.

5. Gently fold in fresh blueberries into the batter.

6. Divide the batter evenly among the muffin cups.

7. Bake for 18-20 minutes or until a toothpick inserted into the center of a muffin comes out clean.

8. Allow the muffins to cool slightly before serving.

Chapter 3: Lunch Recipes

In this chapter, we'll explore a delightful selection of plant-based lunch recipes that are not only incredibly delicious but also packed with wholesome ingredients to nourish your body. From vibrant salads to hearty tacos and comforting soups, these lunch options are designed to cater to your taste buds and provide essential nutrients for your well-being.

Rainbow Veggie and Quinoa Salad with Lemon-Tahini Dressing

Ingredients:

- 1 cup quinoa, rinsed and cooked
- 1 cup cherry tomatoes, halved
- 1 cup cucumber, diced
- 1 cup red bell pepper, thinly sliced
- 1 cup yellow bell pepper, thinly sliced
- 1 cup shredded carrots
- 1/2 cup red onion, thinly sliced
- 1/4 cup fresh parsley, chopped

- 1/4 cup fresh mint leaves, chopped
- 1/4 cup roasted sunflower seeds

Lemon-Tahini Dressing:

- 1/4 cup tahini
- 2 tablespoons fresh lemon juice
- 2 tablespoons water
- 1 tablespoon maple syrup
- 1 clove garlic, minced
- Salt and pepper to taste

Instructions:

1. In a large mixing bowl, combine the cooked quinoa, cherry tomatoes, cucumber, bell peppers, shredded carrots, red onion, parsley, and mint leaves.
2. To prepare the dressing, whisk together the tahini, fresh lemon juice, water, maple syrup, minced garlic, salt, and pepper until smooth.
3. Pour the lemon-tahini dressing over the quinoa and veggies, and toss until well coated.
4. Sprinkle the roasted sunflower seeds on top for added crunch and flavor.

5. Serve the Rainbow Veggie and Quinoa Salad
   chilled, and enjoy a burst of colors and textures in
   every refreshing bite.

Mediterranean Chickpea Salad with Fresh Herbs

Ingredients:

- 2 cups cooked chickpeas (or canned, drained, and rinsed)
- 1 cup cherry tomatoes, halved
- 1 cup cucumber, diced
- 1/2 cup red bell pepper, diced
- 1/2 cup Kalamata olives, pitted and halved
- 1/4 cup red onion, finely chopped
- 1/4 cup fresh parsley, chopped
- 2 tablespoons fresh dill, chopped
- 2 tablespoons fresh lemon juice
- 2 tablespoons extra-virgin olive oil
- 1 clove garlic, minced
- Salt and pepper to taste

Instructions:

1. In a large bowl, combine the cooked chickpeas, cherry tomatoes, cucumber, red bell pepper, Kalamata olives, and red onion.

2. In a separate small bowl, whisk together the fresh parsley, dill, lemon juice, olive oil, minced garlic, salt, and pepper to create the dressing.

3. Drizzle the dressing over the chickpea salad and toss gently to ensure even distribution.

4. Allow the flavors to meld together by refrigerating the salad for at least 30 minutes before serving.

5. Serve the Mediterranean Chickpea Salad as a light and satisfying lunch option or as a side dish for your main course.

Lentil and Vegetable Soup

Ingredients:

- 1 cup green lentils, rinsed and drained
- 1 tablespoon olive oil
- 1 onion, diced
- 2 cloves garlic, minced
- 2 carrots, diced

- 2 celery stalks, diced
- 1 zucchini, diced
- 1 teaspoon ground cumin
- 1 teaspoon ground coriander
- 1/2 teaspoon smoked paprika
- 1/4 teaspoon red pepper flakes (optional)
- 4 cups vegetable broth
- 2 cups water
- 1 can (14 ounces) diced tomatoes
- Salt and pepper to taste
- Fresh parsley for garnish

Instructions:

1. In a large pot, heat the olive oil over medium heat. Add the diced onion and minced garlic, and sauté until the onion becomes translucent.
2. Add the diced carrots, celery, and zucchini to the pot, and continue to sauté for a few more minutes until the vegetables slightly soften.
3. Stir in the ground cumin, ground coriander, smoked paprika, and red pepper flakes (if using) to infuse the soup with aromatic flavors.

4. Add the rinsed lentils, vegetable broth, water, and diced tomatoes to the pot. Bring the mixture to a boil, then reduce the heat and let it simmer for about 20-25 minutes or until the lentils are tender.

5. Season the lentil and vegetable soup with salt and pepper to taste. Garnish with fresh parsley before serving, and relish the heartwarming and nourishing goodness of this comforting lunchtime soup.

Stuffed Bell Peppers with Brown Rice and Lentils

Ingredients:

- 4 large bell peppers (any color)
- 1 cup cooked brown rice
- 1 cup cooked green lentils
- 1 cup diced tomatoes
- 1/2 cup corn kernels (fresh or frozen)
- 1/2 cup black beans (cooked or canned, drained and rinsed)
- 1/2 cup diced red onion
- 2 cloves garlic, minced

- 1 teaspoon ground cumin
- 1 teaspoon chili powder
- 1/2 teaspoon dried oregano
- Salt and pepper to taste
- 1/2 cup vegan shredded cheese (optional)

Instructions:

1. Preheat the oven to 375°F (190°C).
2. Cut the tops off the bell peppers and remove the seeds and membranes.
3. In a large mixing bowl, combine the cooked brown rice, cooked green lentils, diced tomatoes, corn kernels, black beans, diced red onion, minced garlic, ground cumin, chili powder, dried oregano, salt, and pepper. Mix everything well.
4. Stuff the bell peppers with the lentil and rice mixture, pressing down gently to fill them evenly.
5. If desired, sprinkle vegan shredded cheese on top of the stuffed bell peppers for added indulgence.
6. Place the stuffed bell peppers in a baking dish and cover with foil.

7. Bake in the preheated oven for 30 minutes, then remove the foil and bake for an additional 10 minutes to allow the tops to slightly brown.

8. Serve the Stuffed Bell Peppers with Brown Rice and Lentils as a wholesome and hearty lunch option that satisfies both taste and nutritional needs.

Grilled Eggplant and Zucchini Panini with Pesto

Ingredients:

- 1 small eggplant, sliced
- 1 small zucchini, sliced lengthwise
- 1 tablespoon olive oil
- 4 slices whole-grain bread
- 1/4 cup vegan pesto
- 1 cup baby spinach leaves
- 1/2 cup vegan mozzarella cheese, shredded (optional)

Instructions:

1. Preheat a grill or grill pan over medium-high heat.

2. Brush the eggplant and zucchini slices with olive oil, then grill them for 2-3 minutes on each side until they develop grill marks and become tender.

3. Assemble the paninis by spreading a generous amount of vegan pesto on each slice of whole-grain bread.

4. Layer the grilled eggplant and zucchini slices on one side of the bread slices.

5. Top the vegetables with baby spinach leaves and vegan mozzarella cheese (if using).

6. Place the other slice of bread on top to create a sandwich.

7. Heat a panini press or grill pan over medium heat. Place the assembled paninis in the press or grill pan, and cook for 3-4 minutes on each side until the bread is toasted, and the cheese (if using) is melted.

8. Remove the paninis from the heat, slice them in half, and enjoy this delectable combination of grilled veggies and pesto in every bite.

Cauliflower Rice Stir-fry with Tofu and Veggies

Ingredients:

- 1 medium cauliflower head, grated or pulsed into rice-like texture
- 8 ounces firm tofu, drained and cubed
- 1 tablespoon sesame oil
- 2 tablespoons low-sodium soy sauce
- 1 tablespoon rice vinegar
- 1 tablespoon maple syrup
- 2 cloves garlic, minced
- 1 cup broccoli florets
- 1 cup sliced bell peppers (any color)
- 1 cup sliced carrots
- 1 cup snap peas
- 1/2 cup sliced green onions
- 1 tablespoon sesame seeds for garnish

Instructions:

1. In a large skillet or wok, heat the sesame oil over medium-high heat.

2. Add the cubed tofu and cook until lightly browned on all sides. Remove the tofu from the skillet and set aside.

3. In the same skillet, add the minced garlic and sauté for a minute until fragrant.

4. Add the broccoli florets, sliced bell peppers, sliced carrots, and snap peas to the skillet. Stir-fry the veggies for 3-4 minutes until they become tender-crisp.

5. In a small bowl, whisk together the low-sodium soy sauce, rice vinegar, and maple syrup to create the stir-fry sauce.

6. Push the vegetables to one side of the skillet and add the grated cauliflower rice to the other side.

7. Pour the stir-fry sauce over the cauliflower rice and mix everything together to coat the rice and veggies evenly.

8. Add the cooked tofu back into the skillet and toss everything together until well combined.

9. Garnish the Cauliflower Rice Stir-fry with Tofu and Veggies with sliced green onions and sesame seeds

before serving, and relish this light yet flavorful lunch option.

Sweet Potato and Black Bean Tacos

Ingredients:

- 2 medium sweet potatoes, peeled and cubed
- 1 tablespoon olive oil
- 1 teaspoon ground cumin
- 1 teaspoon chili powder
- 1/2 teaspoon paprika
- Salt and pepper to taste
- 8 small corn tortillas
- 1 cup cooked black beans (or canned, drained, and rinsed)
- 1 avocado, sliced
- 1/4 cup diced red onion
- Fresh cilantro leaves for garnish
- Lime wedges for serving

Instructions:

1. Preheat the oven to 400°F (200°C).

2. In a large mixing bowl, toss the sweet potato cubes with olive oil, ground cumin, chili powder, paprika, salt, and pepper until evenly coated.

3. Spread the seasoned sweet potatoes in a single layer on a baking sheet lined with parchment paper.

4. Roast the sweet potatoes in the preheated oven for 20-25 minutes or until they are tender and slightly caramelized, stirring halfway through to ensure even cooking.

5. Warm the corn tortillas on a skillet over medium heat for a minute on each side until they become pliable.

6. To assemble the tacos, spread a spoonful of cooked black beans on each tortilla, then top with the roasted sweet potatoes, sliced avocado, and diced red onion.

7. Garnish the Sweet Potato and Black Bean Tacos with fresh cilantro leaves and serve with lime wedges for squeezing over the tacos before devouring this delightful medley of flavors.

Spinach and Mushroom Quiche with a Chickpea Flour Crust

Ingredients:

Chickpea Flour Crust:

- 1 cup chickpea flour
- 1/4 cup nutritional yeast
- 1/2 teaspoon salt
- 1/4 teaspoon black pepper
- 1/4 teaspoon garlic powder
- 1/4 teaspoon onion powder
- 1/4 teaspoon dried thyme
- 1/4 teaspoon dried rosemary
- 1/4 cup water
- 2 tablespoons olive oil

Spinach and Mushroom Filling:

- 1 tablespoon olive oil
- 1 onion, diced
- 2 cloves garlic, minced
- 8 ounces mushrooms, sliced
- 4 cups fresh spinach leaves

- 1 cup unsweetened plant-based milk (e.g., almond milk, soy milk)
- 3 tablespoons chickpea flour
- 1/4 cup nutritional yeast
- 1/2 teaspoon ground turmeric
- Salt and pepper to taste

Instructions:

1. Preheat the oven to 375°F (190°C).
2. For the chickpea flour crust, in a mixing bowl, whisk together the chickpea flour, nutritional yeast, salt, black pepper, garlic powder, onion powder, dried thyme, and dried rosemary.
3. Add the water and olive oil to the dry ingredients, and stir until a thick, smooth batter forms.
4. Grease a 9-inch pie dish with oil or cooking spray. Pour the chickpea flour batter into the pie dish, and spread it evenly to form the crust.
5. Bake the crust in the preheated oven for 12-15 minutes or until it sets and turns golden brown around the edges.

6. While the crust is baking, prepare the spinach and mushroom filling. In a large skillet, heat olive oil over medium heat.

7. Add the diced onion and minced garlic, and sauté until the onion becomes translucent.

8. Add the sliced mushrooms to the skillet, and cook until they release their moisture and become tender.

9. Stir in the fresh spinach leaves, and cook until the spinach wilts.

10. In a small bowl, whisk together the unsweetened plant-based milk, chickpea flour, nutritional yeast, ground turmeric, salt, and pepper to create the quiche filling.

11. Pour the quiche filling over the sautéed vegetables, and stir to combine.

12. Once the chickpea flour crust is ready, remove it from the oven, and pour the spinach and mushroom filling into the crust.

13. Return the quiche to the oven, and bake for an additional 20-25 minutes until the filling sets.

14. Allow the Spinach and Mushroom Quiche with a Chickpea Flour Crust to cool slightly before slicing

and serving this savory and protein-packed lunch option.

Cucumber and Avocado Sushi Rolls

Ingredients:

- 2 cups sushi rice
- 1/4 cup rice vinegar
- 2 tablespoons sugar
- 1 teaspoon salt
- 4 nori seaweed sheets
- 1 large cucumber, peeled and cut into long strips
- 1 avocado, thinly sliced
- Pickled ginger, for serving
- Wasabi paste, for serving
- Soy sauce, for serving

Instructions:

1. Rinse the sushi rice in a fine-mesh sieve under cold running water until the water runs clear.
2. In a saucepan, combine the rinsed sushi rice with 2 cups of water. Bring to a boil over medium-high heat.

3. Reduce the heat to low, cover the saucepan with a lid, and let the rice simmer for 15-18 minutes or until the rice is cooked and the water is absorbed.

4. In a small bowl, mix the rice vinegar, sugar, and salt until the sugar and salt dissolve.

5. Transfer the cooked rice to a large mixing bowl, and pour the vinegar mixture over the rice. Gently fold the rice with a spatula or rice paddle to combine and evenly distribute the seasoning.

6. Let the seasoned sushi rice cool to room temperature before assembling the sushi rolls.

7. Lay a bamboo sushi rolling mat on a clean surface. Place a nori seaweed sheet shiny side down on the mat.

8. Wet your fingers with water to prevent the rice from sticking, and spread a thin, even layer of sushi rice over the nori sheet, leaving about 1-inch of nori exposed at the top edge.

9. Arrange cucumber strips and avocado slices in a line across the center of the rice-covered nori sheet.

10. Using the bamboo mat, carefully roll the sushi away from you, pressing firmly to shape it into a tight cylinder.
11. Once the roll is complete, wet the exposed edge of the nori sheet with a little water to seal the roll.
12. Repeat the process to create the remaining cucumber and avocado sushi rolls.
13. Use a sharp knife to slice each roll into bite-sized pieces.
14. Serve the Cucumber and Avocado Sushi Rolls with pickled ginger, wasabi paste, and soy sauce for dipping, and savor the fresh and delightful flavors of homemade sushi.

Greek-style Lemon Potatoes with Roasted Asparagus

Ingredients:

- 4 large russet potatoes, peeled and cut into wedges
- 1/4 cup olive oil
- 1/4 cup fresh lemon juice
- 1 teaspoon dried oregano

- 1 teaspoon dried thyme

- 1 teaspoon garlic powder

- Salt and pepper to taste

- 1 bunch asparagus, trimmed

Instructions:

1. Preheat the oven to 400°F (200°C).

2. In a large mixing bowl, combine the potato wedges with olive oil, fresh lemon juice, dried oregano, dried thyme, garlic powder, salt, and pepper. Toss until the potatoes are well coated with the seasoning.

3. Arrange the seasoned potato wedges on a baking sheet lined with parchment paper, leaving some space between the wedges to ensure even cooking.

4. Roast the potatoes in the preheated oven for 30-35 minutes or until they turn golden brown and crispy on the outside, and tender on the inside. Stir the potatoes halfway through the roasting process to ensure even browning.

5. While the potatoes are roasting, prepare the roasted asparagus. Toss the trimmed asparagus with a drizzle of olive oil, salt, and pepper.

6. After removing the potatoes from the oven, place the asparagus on the same baking sheet, and roast them for 8-10 minutes or until they become tender-crisp.

7. Serve the Greek-style Lemon Potatoes with Roasted Asparagus as a delightful lunch option with a burst of Mediterranean flavors that will leave you wanting more.

Chapter 4: Dinner Recipes

In this chapter, we present a delectable collection of plant-based dinner recipes that are not only delicious but also suitable for individuals with diabetic kidney disease. These recipes incorporate a wide array of flavors, textures, and nutrients, making them perfect for promoting health while satisfying your taste buds.

Creamy Vegan Alfredo with Asparagus and Peas

Ingredients:

- 8 oz (225g) whole grain or gluten-free fettuccine
- 1 cup asparagus spears, trimmed and cut into bite-sized pieces
- 1 cup green peas (fresh or frozen)
- 1 cup raw cashews, soaked in water for 4 hours or overnight
- 1/2 cup unsweetened almond milk
- 2 cloves garlic, minced
- 2 tablespoons nutritional yeast

- 1 tablespoon lemon juice
- 1 tablespoon olive oil
- Salt and black pepper to taste
- Fresh parsley for garnish

Instructions:

1. Cook the fettuccine according to the package instructions. In the last 3 minutes of cooking, add the asparagus and peas. Drain and set aside.

2. In a blender, combine the soaked cashews, almond milk, minced garlic, nutritional yeast, lemon juice, and olive oil. Blend until smooth and creamy. Add water if needed to achieve the desired consistency.

3. Heat a large skillet over medium heat. Pour the creamy sauce into the skillet and cook for a few minutes until heated through. Season with salt and black pepper to taste.

4. Add the cooked fettuccine, asparagus, and peas to the skillet. Toss everything together until well coated with the sauce.

5. Serve the Creamy Vegan Alfredo garnished with fresh parsley and additional black pepper if desired.

Eggplant Parmesan with Marinara Sauce and Cashew Cheese

Ingredients:

- 1 large eggplant, sliced into 1/4-inch rounds
- 1 cup whole wheat or gluten-free breadcrumbs
- 1/4 cup nutritional yeast
- 1 teaspoon dried oregano
- 1 teaspoon dried basil
- 1/2 teaspoon garlic powder
- 1/2 teaspoon onion powder
- Salt and black pepper to taste
- 1 cup marinara sauce (store-bought or homemade)
- 1 cup raw cashews, soaked in water for 4 hours or overnight
- 1/2 cup water
- 1 tablespoon lemon juice
- 1/2 teaspoon apple cider vinegar

Instructions:

1. Preheat the oven to 375°F (190°C). Line a baking sheet with parchment paper.

2. In a shallow dish, combine the breadcrumbs,
    nutritional yeast, dried oregano, dried basil, garlic
    powder, onion powder, salt, and black pepper.

3. Dip each eggplant slice into water and then coat
    both sides with the breadcrumb mixture. Place the
    coated slices on the prepared baking sheet.

4. Bake the eggplant slices in the preheated oven for
    25-30 minutes, flipping halfway through, until they
    are golden and crispy.

5. Meanwhile, prepare the cashew cheese by draining
    the soaked cashews and placing them in a blender
    with water, lemon juice, apple cider vinegar, and a
    pinch of salt. Blend until smooth and creamy.

6. In a baking dish, spread a thin layer of marinara
    sauce at the bottom. Arrange a layer of baked
    eggplant slices on top, followed by a layer of
    cashew cheese. Repeat the layers until all
    ingredients are used, finishing with a layer of
    cashew cheese on top.

7. Bake the Eggplant Parmesan in the oven for an
    additional 15-20 minutes until the cheese is slightly
    browned and bubbly.

8. Allow the dish to cool slightly before serving. Enjoy this wholesome Eggplant Parmesan with a side of mixed greens.

Moroccan Chickpea Stew with Couscous

Ingredients:

- 1 tablespoon olive oil
- 1 large onion, chopped
- 3 cloves garlic, minced
- 1 red bell pepper, diced
- 1 yellow bell pepper, diced
- 2 carrots, peeled and diced
- 1 teaspoon ground cumin
- 1 teaspoon ground coriander
- 1/2 teaspoon ground cinnamon
- 1/4 teaspoon cayenne pepper (optional, adjust to taste)
- 1 can (15 oz) diced tomatoes
- 3 cups cooked chickpeas (or 2 cans, drained and rinsed)

- 3 cups vegetable broth

- 1/2 cup dried apricots, chopped

- 1/4 cup raisins

- Salt and black pepper to taste

- 1 cup whole wheat couscous (cooked according to package instructions)

Instructions:

1. In a large pot or Dutch oven, heat the olive oil over medium heat. Add the chopped onion and sauté until softened and translucent.

2. Stir in the minced garlic, diced red and yellow bell peppers, and diced carrots. Cook for a few minutes until the vegetables start to soften.

3. Add the ground cumin, ground coriander, ground cinnamon, and cayenne pepper (if using). Stir well to coat the vegetables with the spices.

4. Pour in the diced tomatoes with their juices, cooked chickpeas, and vegetable broth. Bring the mixture to a boil, then reduce the heat to low and simmer for 15-20 minutes to allow the flavors to meld together.

5. Add the chopped dried apricots and raisins to the stew. Continue to simmer for an additional 5 minutes until the apricots are tender and plump.

6. Season the Moroccan Chickpea Stew with salt and black pepper to taste.

7. Serve the stew over cooked whole wheat couscous, garnishing with fresh cilantro or parsley if desired.

Vegan Mushroom Stroganoff over Brown Rice

Ingredients:

- 2 cups cooked brown rice
- 1 tablespoon olive oil
- 1 onion, finely chopped
- 3 cups sliced mushrooms (button or cremini)
- 2 cloves garlic, minced
- 1 tablespoon all-purpose flour or cornstarch
- 1 cup vegetable broth
- 1 cup unsweetened almond milk
- 2 tablespoons nutritional yeast
- 2 tablespoons soy sauce or tamari

- 1 teaspoon Dijon mustard
- Salt and black pepper to taste
- Fresh parsley for garnish

Instructions:

1. In a large skillet, heat the olive oil over medium heat. Add the chopped onion and sauté until softened and translucent.
2. Add the sliced mushrooms to the skillet and cook until they release their moisture and become tender.
3. Stir in the minced garlic and cook for another minute until fragrant.
4. Sprinkle the flour or cornstarch over the mushrooms and stir to coat evenly.
5. Pour in the vegetable broth and unsweetened almond milk, stirring constantly to avoid lumps. Bring the mixture to a simmer.
6. Reduce the heat to low and add the nutritional yeast, soy sauce or tamari, and Dijon mustard. Stir well to combine all the flavors.

7. Allow the Vegan Mushroom Stroganoff to simmer for a few more minutes until the sauce thickens and the mushrooms are well coated.

8. Season with salt and black pepper to taste.

9. Serve the creamy Mushroom Stroganoff over cooked brown rice, garnished with fresh parsley.

Thai Green Curry with Tofu and Vegetables

Ingredients:

- 1 cup cooked jasmine rice
- 1 tablespoon coconut oil
- 1 small onion, finely chopped
- 2 tablespoons green curry paste (store-bought or homemade)
- 1 can (13.5 oz) coconut milk
- 1 cup vegetable broth
- 1 red bell pepper, sliced
- 1 zucchini, sliced
- 1 cup broccoli florets
- 1 cup firm tofu, cubed

- 1 tablespoon soy sauce or tamari
- 1 tablespoon brown sugar or coconut sugar
- Juice of 1 lime
- Fresh cilantro for garnish

Crushed red pepper flakes (optional, for added spice)

Instructions:

1. In a large wok or skillet, heat the coconut oil over medium heat. Add the chopped onion and sauté until softened and fragrant.
2. Stir in the green curry paste and cook for a minute to release its flavors.
3. Pour in the coconut milk and vegetable broth, stirring well to combine. Bring the mixture to a gentle simmer.
4. Add the sliced red bell pepper, zucchini, broccoli, and tofu to the wok. Cook for about 5-7 minutes or until the vegetables are tender-crisp and the tofu is heated through.

5. Stir in the soy sauce or tamari, brown sugar or coconut sugar, and lime juice. Adjust the seasoning according to your taste preferences.

6. If desired, add some crushed red pepper flakes for extra spiciness.

7. Serve the aromatic Thai Green Curry over cooked jasmine rice, garnishing with fresh cilantro.

Jackfruit and Black Bean Enchiladas

Ingredients:

- 1 can (20 oz) young green jackfruit in brine, drained and rinsed
- 1 tablespoon olive oil
- 1 small onion, finely chopped
- 2 cloves garlic, minced
- 1 teaspoon ground cumin
- 1/2 teaspoon chili powder
- 1/2 teaspoon paprika
- 1 can (15 oz) black beans, drained and rinsed
- 1 cup corn kernels (fresh, frozen, or canned)
- 1 cup enchilada sauce (store-bought or homemade)
- 6-8 small corn tortillas

- 1 cup vegan shredded cheese (cheddar or mozzarella)
- Fresh cilantro for garnish
- Lime wedges for serving

Instructions:

1. Preheat the oven to 375°F (190°C). Grease a baking dish with cooking spray or olive oil.
2. Prepare the jackfruit by shredding it using a fork or your hands, mimicking the texture of pulled pork.
3. In a large skillet, heat the olive oil over medium heat. Add the chopped onion and sauté until softened and translucent.
4. Stir in the minced garlic, ground cumin, chili powder, and paprika. Cook for a minute until the spices become fragrant.
5. Add the shredded jackfruit to the skillet and cook for 5 minutes to allow it to absorb the flavors.
6. Add the black beans and corn kernels to the skillet. Cook for an additional 2-3 minutes until everything is well combined.

7. Pour half of the enchilada sauce into the bottom of the greased baking dish.

8. Warm the corn tortillas in a separate skillet or microwave to make them pliable.

9. Spoon the jackfruit and black bean filling onto each tortilla and roll them up tightly. Place the rolled enchiladas seam-side down in the baking dish.

10. Pour the remaining enchilada sauce over the rolled tortillas, spreading it evenly to cover all the enchiladas.

11. Sprinkle the vegan shredded cheese over the top of the enchiladas.

12. Bake the Jackfruit and Black Bean Enchiladas in the preheated oven for 20-25 minutes until the cheese is melted and bubbly.

13. Garnish the enchiladas with fresh cilantro and serve with lime wedges for added zest.

Chapter 5: Snacks and Appetizers

In this chapter, we'll explore a delightful array of plant-based snacks and appetizers perfect for satisfying your cravings in a healthy and flavorful way. These recipes are designed to please your taste buds while providing essential nutrients to support your well-being.

Baked Sweet Potato Fries with Smoky Paprika Dip

Ingredients:

- 2 large sweet potatoes, peeled and cut into thin fries
- 2 tablespoons olive oil
- 1 teaspoon smoked paprika
- 1/2 teaspoon garlic powder
- 1/2 teaspoon onion powder
- Salt and pepper to taste

Smoky Paprika Dip:

- 1/2 cup vegan mayonnaise
- 1 tablespoon lemon juice

- 1 teaspoon smoked paprika
- 1/2 teaspoon cayenne pepper
- Salt and pepper to taste

Instructions:

1. Preheat your oven to 425°F (220°C) and line a baking sheet with parchment paper.
2. In a large bowl, toss the sweet potato fries with olive oil, smoked paprika, garlic powder, onion powder, salt, and pepper until evenly coated.
3. Spread the seasoned fries in a single layer on the prepared baking sheet.
4. Bake for 20-25 minutes or until the fries are crispy and golden brown, flipping them halfway through the baking time for even cooking.
5. While the fries are baking, prepare the smoky paprika dip by whisking together all the dip ingredients in a small bowl.
6. Serve the baked sweet potato fries hot with the smoky paprika dip on the side.

Zucchini and Carrot Fritters with Mint Yogurt Sauce

Ingredients:

- 2 medium zucchinis, grated
- 2 medium carrots, grated
- 1/2 cup chickpea flour
- 2 tablespoons nutritional yeast
- 1 teaspoon ground cumin
- 1/2 teaspoon baking powder
- Salt and pepper to taste
- 2 tablespoons chopped fresh parsley
- 2 tablespoons chopped fresh dill
- Olive oil for frying

Mint Yogurt Sauce:

- 1 cup dairy-free yogurt
- 2 tablespoons fresh mint leaves, finely chopped
- 1 tablespoon lemon juice
- 1 garlic clove, minced
- Salt and pepper to taste

Instructions:

1. Place the grated zucchini and carrots in a colander
    and sprinkle with a pinch of salt. Allow them to sit
    for 10 minutes, then squeeze out the excess
    moisture using a clean kitchen towel.

2. In a large bowl, combine the squeezed zucchini and
    carrots with chickpea flour, nutritional yeast,
    ground cumin, baking powder, salt, pepper,
    chopped parsley, and dill. Mix well to form a thick
    batter.

3. Heat a thin layer of olive oil in a non-stick skillet
    over medium heat.

4. Spoon the fritter batter into the hot skillet, shaping
    each fritter with a spoon. Cook for 3-4 minutes on
    each side or until golden brown and crispy.

5. For the mint yogurt sauce, mix all the sauce
    ingredients in a small bowl until well combined.

6. Serve the zucchini and carrot fritters warm with a
    dollop of mint yogurt sauce on top.

Edamame with Sea Salt and Lime

Ingredients:

- 2 cups frozen edamame, thawed

- Sea salt to taste

- 1 lime, cut into wedges

Instructions:

1. Bring a pot of water to a boil and add the thawed edamame. Cook for 2-3 minutes until tender.
2. Drain the edamame and transfer them to a serving bowl.
3. Sprinkle sea salt over the edamame and squeeze fresh lime juice on top.
4. Toss to coat the edamame evenly with the seasoning.
5. Serve the edamame warm as a nutritious and refreshing snack.

Spicy Buffalo Cauliflower Bites with Vegan Ranch Dip

Ingredients:

- 1 medium head of cauliflower, cut into bite-sized florets

- 1 cup almond milk

- 3/4 cup chickpea flour

- 1 teaspoon garlic powder

- 1 teaspoon onion powder

- 1/2 teaspoon smoked paprika

- 1/4 teaspoon cayenne pepper (adjust to your spice preference)

- Salt and pepper to taste

Buffalo Sauce:

- 1/2 cup hot sauce of your choice

- 2 tablespoons melted vegan butter

Vegan Ranch Dip:

- 1 cup vegan mayonnaise

- 1/4 cup unsweetened almond milk

- 1 tablespoon fresh dill, chopped

- 1 tablespoon fresh parsley, chopped

- 1 clove garlic, minced

- 1 tablespoon lemon juice

- Salt and pepper to taste

Instructions:

1. Preheat your oven to 450°F (230°C) and line a baking sheet with parchment paper.
2. In a large bowl, whisk together almond milk, chickpea flour, garlic powder, onion powder, smoked paprika, cayenne pepper, salt, and pepper until you get a smooth batter.
3. Dip each cauliflower floret into the batter, coating it completely, and place it on the prepared baking sheet.
4. Bake for 20-25 minutes or until the cauliflower is crispy and golden brown.
5. While the cauliflower is baking, prepare the buffalo sauce by mixing the hot sauce and melted vegan butter in a bowl.
6. Toss the baked cauliflower in the buffalo sauce until evenly coated.
7. For the vegan ranch dip, combine all the dip ingredients in a small bowl and mix well.
8. Serve the spicy buffalo cauliflower bites with the vegan ranch dip on the side for a satisfying and flavorful snack.

Guacamole with Baked Tortilla Chips

Ingredients:

- 3 ripe avocados, peeled and pitted
- 1/4 cup finely chopped red onion
- 1/4 cup diced tomatoes
- 2 tablespoons chopped fresh cilantro
- 1 tablespoon fresh lime juice
- 1 small jalapeño pepper, seeded and finely chopped (optional for spice)
- Salt and pepper to taste

Baked Tortilla Chips:

- 6-8 whole wheat tortillas
- Olive oil spray
- Salt to taste

Instructions:

1. In a medium bowl, mash the avocados with a fork until you achieve your desired guacamole consistency.

2. Add the chopped red onion, diced tomatoes, cilantro, lime juice, and jalapeño (if using) to the mashed avocados.

3. Season the guacamole with salt and pepper, and mix well until all the ingredients are combined.

4. For the baked tortilla chips, preheat your oven to 350°F (175°C).

5. Cut each whole wheat tortilla into triangles or desired shapes.

6. Arrange the tortilla pieces on a baking sheet lined with parchment paper.

7. Lightly spray the tortilla pieces with olive oil and sprinkle salt over them.

8. Bake the tortilla chips for 10-12 minutes or until they are crispy and golden brown.

9. Serve the guacamole with the freshly baked tortilla chips for a classic and healthy snack.

Stuffed Mushrooms with Quinoa and Spinach

Ingredients:

- 12 large white mushrooms, stems removed and reserved
- 1 cup cooked quinoa
- 1 cup fresh spinach, chopped
- 1/4 cup diced red bell pepper
- 2 cloves garlic, minced
- 2 tablespoons nutritional yeast
- 1 tablespoon olive oil
- Salt and pepper to taste
- 2 tablespoons chopped fresh parsley

Instructions:

1. Preheat your oven to 375°F (190°C) and line a baking sheet with parchment paper.
2. Clean the mushroom caps and set them aside. Finely chop the reserved mushroom stems.
3. In a skillet, heat olive oil over medium heat and sauté the chopped mushroom stems, diced red bell pepper, and minced garlic until softened.

4. Add the chopped spinach to the skillet and cook until wilted.

5. In a bowl, combine the cooked quinoa, sautéed vegetables, nutritional yeast, salt, pepper, and chopped parsley. Mix well.

6. Stuff each mushroom cap with the quinoa and spinach mixture, pressing gently to pack it.

7. Arrange the stuffed mushrooms on the prepared baking sheet.

8. Bake for 15-20 minutes or until the mushrooms are tender and slightly browned.

9. Serve the stuffed mushrooms warm as an appetizing and nutrient-packed snack.

Cucumber, Radish, and Vegan Cream Cheese Tea Sandwiches

Ingredients:

- 8 slices whole grain bread
- 1 cup vegan cream cheese
- 1 cucumber, thinly sliced
- 6-8 radishes, thinly sliced

- 2 tablespoons fresh dill, chopped

- Salt and pepper to taste

Instructions:

1. Trim the crusts off the whole grain bread slices to form neat squares or rectangles for tea sandwiches.

2. Spread a generous layer of vegan cream cheese on one side of each bread slice.

3. On half of the bread slices, arrange the cucumber and radish slices in an even layer.

4. Sprinkle chopped fresh dill, salt, and pepper over the cucumber and radish slices.

5. Top with the remaining bread slices with the cream cheese side facing down, creating sandwich pairs.

6. Press the sandwiches together gently, and if desired, cut them into smaller, bite-sized tea sandwiches.

7. Serve the cucumber, radish, and vegan cream cheese tea sandwiches as a delightful and elegant appetizer for gatherings or afternoon tea.

Roasted Chickpeas with Rosemary and Sea Salt

Ingredients:

- 2 cups cooked chickpeas (or 1 can, drained and rinsed)
- 2 tablespoons olive oil
- 1 tablespoon chopped fresh rosemary
- 1/2 teaspoon garlic powder
- 1/2 teaspoon onion powder
- 1/2 teaspoon smoked paprika
- Sea salt to taste

Instructions:

1. Preheat your oven to 400°F (200°C) and line a baking sheet with parchment paper.
2. In a bowl, toss the cooked chickpeas with olive oil, chopped rosemary, garlic powder, onion powder, smoked paprika, and sea salt until the chickpeas are evenly coated.
3. Spread the seasoned chickpeas on the prepared baking sheet in a single layer.

4. Roast the chickpeas in the preheated oven for 25-30 minutes or until they are crispy and golden brown.

5. Allow the roasted chickpeas to cool slightly before serving.

6. Enjoy the flavorful and crunchy roasted chickpeas as a nutritious and satisfying snack.

Salsa Verde with Homemade Pita Chips

Ingredients:

- 1 cup fresh cilantro leaves
- 1 cup fresh parsley leaves
- 1 clove garlic
- 1 small jalapeño pepper, seeded
- 1/4 cup chopped red onion
- 1 tablespoon lime juice
- 2 tablespoons olive oil
- Salt and pepper to taste

Homemade Pita Chips:

- 4 whole wheat pita bread rounds

- Olive oil spray
- Salt to taste

Instructions:

1. For the salsa verde, combine the cilantro, parsley, garlic, jalapeño, red onion, lime juice, olive oil, salt, and pepper in a food processor.
2. Pulse the ingredients until you get a smooth and flavorful green sauce. Adjust the seasoning to your taste preference.
3. Transfer the salsa verde to a serving bowl.
4. For the homemade pita chips, preheat your oven to 375°F (190°C).
5. Cut each whole wheat pita bread round into triangles or desired shapes.
6. Arrange the pita pieces on a baking sheet lined with parchment paper.
7. Lightly spray the pita chips with olive oil and sprinkle salt over them.
8. Bake the pita chips for 8-10 minutes or until they are crispy and golden brown.

9. Serve the refreshing salsa verde with the freshly baked homemade pita chips for a zesty and crunchy snack.

Marinated Olives and Artichoke Hearts

Ingredients:

- 1 cup mixed olives (green and black), pitted
- 1 cup marinated artichoke hearts, drained
- 2 tablespoons extra-virgin olive oil
- 2 cloves garlic, thinly sliced
- 1 teaspoon dried oregano
- 1/2 teaspoon red pepper flakes (adjust to your spice preference)
- Zest of 1 lemon
- Fresh parsley for garnish

Instructions:

1. In a mixing bowl, combine the mixed olives and drained marinated artichoke hearts.

2. In a small saucepan, heat the extra-virgin olive oil over low heat.

3. Add the thinly sliced garlic to the warm oil and cook for 1-2 minutes until fragrant.

4. Stir in the dried oregano and red pepper flakes, and cook for an additional 1-2 minutes.

5. Pour the warm oil mixture over the olives and artichoke hearts.

6. Add the lemon zest to the bowl and toss all the ingredients together until the olives and artichoke hearts are evenly coated in the marinade.

7. Cover the bowl and let the flavors marinate for at least 30 minutes before serving.

8. Garnish with fresh parsley before serving the marinated olives and artichoke hearts as a delectable and aromatic appetizer.

Chapter 6: Desserts

In this chapter, we will explore a delectable array of plant-based desserts that are not only satisfyingly sweet but also packed with wholesome ingredients. These guilt-free treats will cater to your sweet tooth while ensuring you stay on track with your health goals.

Chocolate Avocado Mousse

Ingredients:

- 2 ripe avocados
- 1/4 cup unsweetened cocoa powder
- 1/4 cup pure maple syrup
- 1/4 cup almond milk
- 1 teaspoon vanilla extract
- Pinch of salt
- Fresh berries for garnish (optional)

Instructions:

1. Cut the avocados in half, remove the pit, and scoop out the flesh into a blender or food processor.

2. Add the cocoa powder, maple syrup, almond milk, vanilla extract, and a pinch of salt to the blender.

3. Blend the mixture on high until it becomes smooth and creamy, scraping down the sides if needed.

4. Transfer the mousse into serving cups or bowls.

5. Chill the mousse in the refrigerator for at least 30 minutes before serving.

6. Garnish with fresh berries if desired, and enjoy this velvety chocolate indulgence guilt-free!

Berry Crisp with Oat and Almond Topping

Ingredients:

- 2 cups mixed fresh or frozen berries (blueberries, raspberries, strawberries, etc.)
- 1 tablespoon lemon juice
- 1/4 cup pure maple syrup
- 1/2 cup rolled oats
- 1/4 cup almond flour
- 1/4 cup sliced almonds
- 2 tablespoons coconut oil, melted

- 1/2 teaspoon ground cinnamon
- Pinch of salt

Instructions:

1. Preheat your oven to 350°F (175°C) and lightly grease a baking dish.
2. In a mixing bowl, toss the mixed berries with lemon juice and 2 tablespoons of maple syrup until coated.
3. Spread the berry mixture evenly in the greased baking dish.
4. In another bowl, combine the rolled oats, almond flour, sliced almonds, melted coconut oil, remaining maple syrup, ground cinnamon, and a pinch of salt. Mix until crumbly.
5. Sprinkle the oat and almond mixture over the berries in the baking dish.
6. Bake in the preheated oven for 25-30 minutes or until the topping turns golden brown and the berries are bubbling.
7. Let it cool slightly before serving. Enjoy this warm, comforting berry crisp on its own or with a scoop of your favorite plant-based ice cream!

Chia Seed and Mixed Fruit Parfait

Ingredients:

- 1/4 cup chia seeds
- 1 cup unsweetened almond milk
- 2 cups mixed fresh fruits (mango, kiwi, pineapple, etc.), diced
- 1 tablespoon pure maple syrup
- 1/4 cup granola (preferably without added sugar)
- Fresh mint leaves for garnish (optional)

Instructions:

1. In a bowl, whisk together the chia seeds and almond milk. Cover the bowl and refrigerate for at least 2 hours or overnight, allowing the chia seeds to swell and create a pudding-like consistency.
2. In a separate bowl, toss the mixed fresh fruits with maple syrup until lightly coated.
3. Assemble the parfait by layering the chia seed pudding, mixed fruits, and granola in serving glasses or jars.

4. Repeat the layers until the ingredients are used up, finishing with a layer of mixed fruits and a sprinkle of granola on top.

5. Garnish with fresh mint leaves if desired.

6. Serve chilled and relish the delightful blend of textures and flavors in this wholesome parfait.

Vegan Lemon Bars with Almond Crust

Ingredients:

- 1 cup almond flour
- 1/4 cup coconut flour
- 1/4 cup coconut oil, melted
- 3 tablespoons pure maple syrup
- 1/4 teaspoon salt
- 1 cup silken tofu
- 1/2 cup fresh lemon juice
- Zest of 1 lemon
- 1/2 cup powdered sugar for dusting

Instructions:

1. Preheat your oven to 350°F (175°C) and grease an 8x8-inch baking dish.
2. In a bowl, mix the almond flour, coconut flour, melted coconut oil, maple syrup, and salt until a dough forms.
3. Press the dough into the bottom of the greased baking dish to form the crust.
4. Bake the crust in the preheated oven for 12-15 minutes or until golden brown. Set it aside to cool.
5. In a blender or food processor, blend the silken tofu, fresh lemon juice, and lemon zest until smooth.
6. Pour the lemon mixture over the cooled crust and spread it evenly.
7. Bake in the oven for an additional 15-20 minutes or until the lemon filling is set.
8. Allow the lemon bars to cool completely in the baking dish before cutting them into squares.
9. Dust the tops of the lemon bars with powdered sugar for an elegant touch.
10. Savor the tangy goodness of these vegan lemon bars that strike a perfect balance between sweet and sour.

Baked Apples with Cinnamon and Maple Syrup

Ingredients:

- 4 large apples (such as Granny Smith or Honeycrisp)
- 2 tablespoons coconut oil, melted
- 2 tablespoons pure maple syrup
- 1 teaspoon ground cinnamon
- Pinch of nutmeg (optional)

Instructions:

1. Preheat your oven to 375°F (190°C) and line a baking sheet with parchment paper.
2. Cut the tops off the apples and use a spoon or melon baller to scoop out the cores, leaving the bottoms intact to create a well for the filling.
3. In a small bowl, mix the melted coconut oil, maple syrup, ground cinnamon, and nutmeg (if using) until well combined.
4. Brush the mixture over the outside and inside of the apples, ensuring they are coated evenly.

5. Place the apples on the prepared baking sheet and bake in the preheated oven for 25-30 minutes or until the apples are tender.

6. Remove the apples from the oven and let them cool slightly before serving.

7. Drizzle any remaining cinnamon and maple syrup mixture over the baked apples for extra flavor.

8. Relish these warm, spiced baked apples as a comforting dessert or serve them with a scoop of dairy-free vanilla ice cream.

Coconut Mango Rice Pudding

Ingredients:

- 1 cup white rice (jasmine or basmati)
- 2 cups coconut milk (full-fat for creaminess)
- 1/4 cup pure maple syrup
- 1 cup diced ripe mango
- 1/4 cup shredded coconut (unsweetened)
- 1 teaspoon vanilla extract
- Pinch of salt

Instructions:

1. Rinse the rice under cold water until the water runs
    clear.
2. In a medium-sized saucepan, combine the rinsed
    rice, coconut milk, maple syrup, and a pinch of salt.
3. Bring the mixture to a boil over medium-high heat,
    stirring occasionally.
4. Once it boils, reduce the heat to low, cover the
    saucepan with a lid, and let it simmer for 20-25
    minutes or until the rice is cooked and the mixture
    has thickened, stirring occasionally.
5. Remove the saucepan from the heat and stir in the
    vanilla extract.
6. Let the rice pudding cool to room temperature.
7. In serving bowls, layer the rice pudding with diced
    mango and shredded coconut.
8. Chill the coconut mango rice pudding in the
    refrigerator for at least 1 hour before serving.
9. Indulge in the tropical flavors of coconut and
    mango in this creamy and satisfying rice pudding.

Pumpkin Spice Energy Bites

Ingredients:

- 1 cup rolled oats
- 1/2 cup canned pumpkin puree
- 1/4 cup almond butter
- 1/4 cup ground flaxseed
- 1/4 cup pure maple syrup
- 1 teaspoon pumpkin pie spice (a mix of cinnamon, nutmeg, ginger, and cloves)
- 1/2 cup chopped walnuts
- 1/4 cup dairy-free chocolate chips (optional)

Instructions:

1. In a large mixing bowl, combine the rolled oats, pumpkin puree, almond butter, ground flaxseed, maple syrup, and pumpkin pie spice.
2. Mix the ingredients until well combined, forming a sticky dough.
3. Fold in the chopped walnuts and dairy-free chocolate chips, if using.
4. Cover the bowl and refrigerate the dough for at least 30 minutes to firm up.

5. Once chilled, remove the dough from the refrigerator and roll it into bite-sized balls using your hands.

6. Place the energy bites on a parchment-lined plate or baking sheet.

7. Refrigerate the energy bites for an additional 15-20 minutes to set.

8. Store the pumpkin spice energy bites in an airtight container in the refrigerator for a quick and energizing snack on-the-go.

Chocolate Chip Chickpea Blondies

Ingredients:

- 1 can (15 ounces) chickpeas (garbanzo beans), drained and rinsed
- 1/2 cup almond butter
- 1/4 cup pure maple syrup
- 2 teaspoons vanilla extract
- 1/2 cup almond flour
- 1/2 teaspoon baking powder
- Pinch of salt
- 1/3 cup dairy-free chocolate chips

Instructions:

1. Preheat your oven to 350°F (175°C) and line an 8x8-inch baking dish with parchment paper.

2. In a food processor, blend the drained chickpeas, almond butter, maple syrup, and vanilla extract until smooth and creamy.

3. Add the almond flour, baking powder, and a pinch of salt to the food processor. Pulse until the ingredients are well combined.

4. Fold in the dairy-free chocolate chips into the chickpea batter.

5. Pour the batter into the prepared baking dish, spreading it out evenly.

6. Bake in the preheated oven for 25-30 minutes or until the edges turn golden brown and a toothpick inserted into the center comes out clean.

7. Let the blondies cool in the baking dish for 10-15 minutes before transferring them to a wire rack to cool completely.

8. Cut the cooled blondies into squares and savor the surprising richness and fudgy texture of these delightful chocolate chip chickpea blondies.

Vegan Carrot Cake with Cashew Cream Frosting

Ingredients:

For the Carrot Cake:

- 2 cups grated carrots
- 1 cup almond flour
- 1 cup whole wheat flour
- 1 cup coconut sugar
- 1/2 cup unsweetened applesauce
- 1/2 cup coconut oil, melted
- 1/2 cup crushed pineapple, drained
- 1/4 cup chopped walnuts or pecans
- 1/4 cup raisins (optional)
- 2 teaspoons baking powder
- 1 teaspoon baking soda
- 1 teaspoon ground cinnamon
- 1/2 teaspoon ground ginger
- 1/4 teaspoon ground nutmeg
- Pinch of salt

For the Cashew Cream Frosting:

- 1 cup raw cashews, soaked in water for at least 4 hours
- 1/4 cup coconut cream
- 1/4 cup pure maple syrup
- 1 teaspoon vanilla extract
- 1 tablespoon lemon juice
- Pinch of salt

Instructions:

For the Carrot Cake:

1. Preheat your oven to 350°F (175°C) and grease an 8-inch round cake pan.
2. In a large mixing bowl, whisk together the almond flour, whole wheat flour, coconut sugar, baking powder, baking soda, ground cinnamon, ground ginger, ground nutmeg, and a pinch of salt.
3. In another bowl, combine the grated carrots, unsweetened applesauce, melted coconut oil, crushed pineapple, chopped walnuts or pecans, and raisins (if using).
4. Fold the wet carrot mixture into the dry flour mixture until well combined.

5. Pour the cake batter into the prepared cake pan and spread it out evenly.

6. Bake in the preheated oven for 35-40 minutes or until a toothpick inserted into the center comes out clean.

7. Remove the carrot cake from the oven and let it cool completely in the pan before frosting.

For the Cashew Cream Frosting:

1. Drain the soaked cashews and rinse them under cold water.

2. In a high-speed blender or food processor, blend the soaked cashews, coconut cream, pure maple syrup, vanilla extract, lemon juice, and a pinch of salt until creamy and smooth.

3. Transfer the cashew cream frosting into a bowl and refrigerate for 30 minutes to firm up slightly.

Assembling the Vegan Carrot Cake:

1. Once the carrot cake has cooled, remove it from the cake pan and place it on a serving platter or cake stand.

2. Spread the cashew cream frosting generously over the top of the carrot cake, creating swirls or patterns with a spatula for an elegant touch.

3. Optionally, garnish the cake with additional chopped nuts, grated carrots, or edible flowers.

4. Slice and serve this delightful vegan carrot cake to revel in the perfect harmony of flavors and textures.

Frozen Banana and Berry Popsicles

Ingredients:

- 2 ripe bananas
- 1 cup mixed fresh berries (blueberries, strawberries, raspberries, etc.)
- 1 cup unsweetened almond milk
- 1 tablespoon pure maple syrup (optional)
- 1/4 teaspoon pure vanilla extract

Instructions:

1. In a blender, combine the ripe bananas, mixed berries, unsweetened almond milk, pure maple syrup (if using), and pure vanilla extract.

2. Blend the mixture until smooth and well combined.

3. Pour the berry and banana mixture into popsicle molds, leaving a little space at the top for expansion.

4. Insert popsicle sticks into each mold.

5. Freeze the popsicles in the freezer for at least 4 hours or until completely frozen.

6. To remove the popsicles from the molds, run warm water over the outside of the molds for a few seconds to loosen them.

7. Delight in these refreshing and naturally sweet frozen banana and berry popsicles as a wholesome and cooling treat.

Chapter 7: Smoothies

In this chapter, we will delve into the delightful world of smoothies, presenting you with unique and scrumptious recipes that are not only delicious but also packed with essential nutrients to support your health and well-being.

Green Goddess Smoothie with Kale and Pineapple

Ingredients:

- 1 cup fresh kale leaves, stems removed
- 1 cup ripe pineapple chunks
- 1 ripe banana
- 1/2 cucumber, peeled and chopped
- 1 tablespoon fresh lemon juice
- 1/2 cup coconut water
- 1/2 cup almond milk
- Ice cubes (optional)

Instructions:

1. In a blender, combine the kale, pineapple, banana, cucumber, lemon juice, coconut water, and almond milk.

2. Blend on high speed until the mixture is smooth and creamy.

3. If you prefer a colder smoothie, add a few ice cubes and blend again until well incorporated.

4. Pour into a glass and enjoy the refreshing goodness of this green goddess smoothie.

Blueberry Almond Smoothie with Flaxseed

Ingredients:

- 1 cup frozen blueberries
- 1 ripe banana
- 1/4 cup almond butter
- 1 tablespoon ground flaxseed
- 1 cup unsweetened almond milk
- 1/2 teaspoon pure vanilla extract
- Honey or maple syrup (optional, for sweetness)

Instructions:

1. Combine the frozen blueberries, ripe banana, almond butter, ground flaxseed, almond milk, and vanilla extract in a blender.
2. Blend until all the ingredients are well combined and the smoothie has a creamy texture.
3. Taste the smoothie and add honey or maple syrup if you prefer a sweeter flavor.
4. Pour into a glass, garnish with a few blueberries if desired, and savor the delightful taste of blueberry and almond in every sip.

Mango and Coconut Smoothie with Turmeric

Ingredients:

- 1 cup ripe mango chunks
- 1/2 cup coconut milk
- 1/2 cup coconut water
- 1 teaspoon fresh turmeric root, grated (or 1/2 teaspoon ground turmeric)
- 1 tablespoon fresh lime juice

- 1 tablespoon shredded coconut (optional, for garnish)

Instructions:

1. In a blender, combine the mango chunks, coconut milk, coconut water, grated turmeric, and lime juice.
2. Blend until the mixture becomes smooth and creamy.
3. Pour the smoothie into a glass and top with shredded coconut for an extra tropical touch.
4. Take a sip and be transported to a sunny beach with the delightful flavors of mango and coconut dancing on your taste buds.

Spinach and Banana Smoothie with Chia Seeds

Ingredients:

- 2 cups fresh spinach leaves
- 2 ripe bananas

- 1 cup unsweetened soy milk (or any plant-based milk of your choice)
- 1 tablespoon chia seeds
- 1 teaspoon honey or agave syrup (optional, for sweetness)

Instructions:

1. Place the fresh spinach leaves, ripe bananas, soy milk, and chia seeds in a blender.
2. Blend until the ingredients are well incorporated and the smoothie is creamy.
3. If you prefer a sweeter taste, add honey or agave syrup and blend again to combine.
4. Pour the green goodness into a glass, and with each sip, revel in the nourishment of this spinach and banana smoothie.

Chocolate Peanut Butter Protein Smoothie

Ingredients:

- 2 tablespoons unsweetened cocoa powder

- 2 tablespoons natural peanut butter

- 1 ripe banana

- 1 cup unsweetened almond milk

- 1/2 cup silken tofu (for added creaminess and protein)

- 1 tablespoon maple syrup (optional, for sweetness)

- Ice cubes (optional)

Instructions:

1. Combine the unsweetened cocoa powder, natural peanut butter, ripe banana, almond milk, silken tofu, and maple syrup (if using) in a blender.

2. Blend until all the ingredients are thoroughly mixed and the smoothie has a rich, chocolaty flavor.

3. Add ice cubes for a cooler and thicker texture, then blend again until well combined.

4. Pour the chocolate peanut butter protein smoothie into a glass, and take pleasure in the harmonious blend of chocolate and peanut butter in each sip.

Raspberry and Beet Smoothie with Hemp Seeds

Ingredients:

- 1 cup fresh or frozen raspberries
- 1 small cooked beet, peeled and chopped
- 1 cup coconut water
- 1 tablespoon hemp seeds
- 1 tablespoon fresh lemon juice
- 1 teaspoon honey or agave syrup (optional, for sweetness)

Instructions:

1. Place the raspberries, cooked beet, coconut water, hemp seeds, and lemon juice in a blender.
2. Blend until the mixture is velvety smooth and has a vibrant pink hue.
3. Taste the smoothie and add honey or agave syrup if you desire a touch of sweetness.
4. Pour into a glass, and with each sip, savor the delightful fusion of raspberry and beet flavors complemented by the nutty essence of hemp seeds.

Tropical Turmeric Smoothie with Ginger and Mango

Ingredients:

- 1 cup ripe mango chunks
- 1 small ripe banana
- 1/2 cup fresh orange juice
- 1/2 cup coconut water
- 1 teaspoon fresh turmeric root, grated (or 1/2 teaspoon ground turmeric)
- 1/2 teaspoon fresh ginger, grated
- Ice cubes (optional)

Instructions:

1. In a blender, combine the mango chunks, ripe banana, orange juice, coconut water, grated turmeric, and grated ginger.
2. Blend until all the ingredients are well blended and the smoothie has a luscious texture.
3. For a cooler smoothie, add ice cubes and blend again until thoroughly mixed.

4. Pour the tropical turmeric smoothie into a glass, close your eyes, and allow the flavors of mango and ginger to transport you to a sunny paradise.

Creamy Avocado and Spinach Smoothie

Ingredients:

- 1 ripe avocado, pitted and peeled
- 2 cups fresh spinach leaves
- 1 cup unsweetened almond milk
- 1 tablespoon fresh lime juice
- 1 tablespoon honey or agave syrup (optional, for sweetness)

Instructions:

1. Combine the ripe avocado, fresh spinach leaves, almond milk, and lime juice in a blender.
2. Blend until the mixture turns smooth and creamy, with a lovely green hue.
3. If you prefer a touch of sweetness, add honey or agave syrup and blend again to incorporate.

4. Pour the creamy avocado and spinach smoothie into a glass, and relish the velvety goodness of this nourishing treat.

Orange and Carrot Smoothie with Vanilla

Ingredients:

- 2 large carrots, peeled and chopped
- 1 large orange, peeled and segmented
- 1 cup coconut water
- 1/2 teaspoon pure vanilla extract
- 1 tablespoon fresh lemon juice
- Ice cubes (optional)

Instructions:

1. Place the chopped carrots, orange segments, coconut water, vanilla extract, and lemon juice in a blender.
2. Blend until the ingredients form a smooth and vibrant orange concoction.

3. If you desire a chilled smoothie, add ice cubes and blend again until well combined.

4. Pour the invigorating orange and carrot smoothie into a glass, and let the zesty flavors of citrus and the earthiness of carrots tantalize your taste buds.

Cherry and Almond Smoothie with Cacao Nibs

Ingredients:

- 1 cup frozen cherries
- 1 cup unsweetened almond milk
- 1 tablespoon almond butter
- 1 tablespoon cacao nibs
- 1 teaspoon honey or maple syrup (optional, for sweetness)

Instructions:

1. In a blender, combine the frozen cherries, almond milk, almond butter, and cacao nibs.

2. Blend until the smoothie becomes velvety and the cherries impart their rich red color.

3. Taste the smoothie and add honey or maple syrup
    for a sweeter taste, if desired.

4. Pour the delightful cherry and almond smoothie into
    a glass, and let the bursts of cherry flavor and the
    crunch of cacao nibs transport you to a moment of
    pure bliss.

CONCLUSION

As we draw the curtains on this extensive journey through "Plant-based Recipes for Diabetic Kidney Disease," we find ourselves at a pivotal moment of reflection and empowerment. Throughout this comprehensive guide, we have explored the remarkable potential of a plant-based lifestyle in managing diabetic kidney disease, uncovering a world of flavors, textures, and nourishment that not only cater to the taste buds but also nurture the body and soul.

By now, you have undoubtedly grasped the significance of adopting a plant-based diet, particularly when faced with the challenges of diabetic kidney disease. The amalgamation of wholesome fruits, vibrant vegetables, hearty legumes, and nourishing grains offers a multitude of benefits that extend beyond glycemic control and kidney health. Embracing this lifestyle has the power to strengthen your overall well-being, uplift your energy levels, and even contribute positively to the environment.

As you embark on this adventure, remember that a plant-based diet is not solely about the food on your plate; it is a holistic lifestyle that encompasses mindfulness, physical activity, and emotional well-being. Engage in regular exercise that brings you joy, practice meditation or yoga to center your mind, and surround yourself with positive influences that uplift your spirits.

Thank you for accompanying us on this enlightening journey. May your future be adorned with vibrant flavors, abundant health, and a heart brimming with joy. Here's to a radiant and flourishing plant-based life, celebrating the wonders it bestows upon you and those around you.

Wishing you the very best on your ongoing quest for wellness and happiness.